FIRST HAND
COMMUNITY
NURSING

FIRST HAND
COMMUNITY
NURSING

Carmen Alicea, RN, MSN, WCC

Library of Congress Control Number:		2012923522
ISBN:	Hardcover	978-1-4797-6593-5
	Softcover	978-1-4797-6592-8
	Ebook	978-1-4797-6594-2

This book was printed in the United States of America.

Rev. date 03/29/2013

To order additional copies of this book, contact:
Xlibris LLC
1-888-795-4274
www.Xlibris.com
Orders@Xlibris.com
118394

This book is to recognize community nurses who provide nursing care in a home setting. Your professional challenges in the community do not go unrecognized.

ACKNOWLEDGMENTS

My personal and sincere thanks to the following:

Dominica Alicea—Without your encouragement and support, this book would have not been possible.

Luis Ojeda—Thank you for believing in me and holding up the fort during my absence.

Carmela Aponte—Thank you for your unique support, which made me stronger.

Special thanks to all who believed in me, who, in some unique way, played a special role in encouraging me to share my community nursing experience.

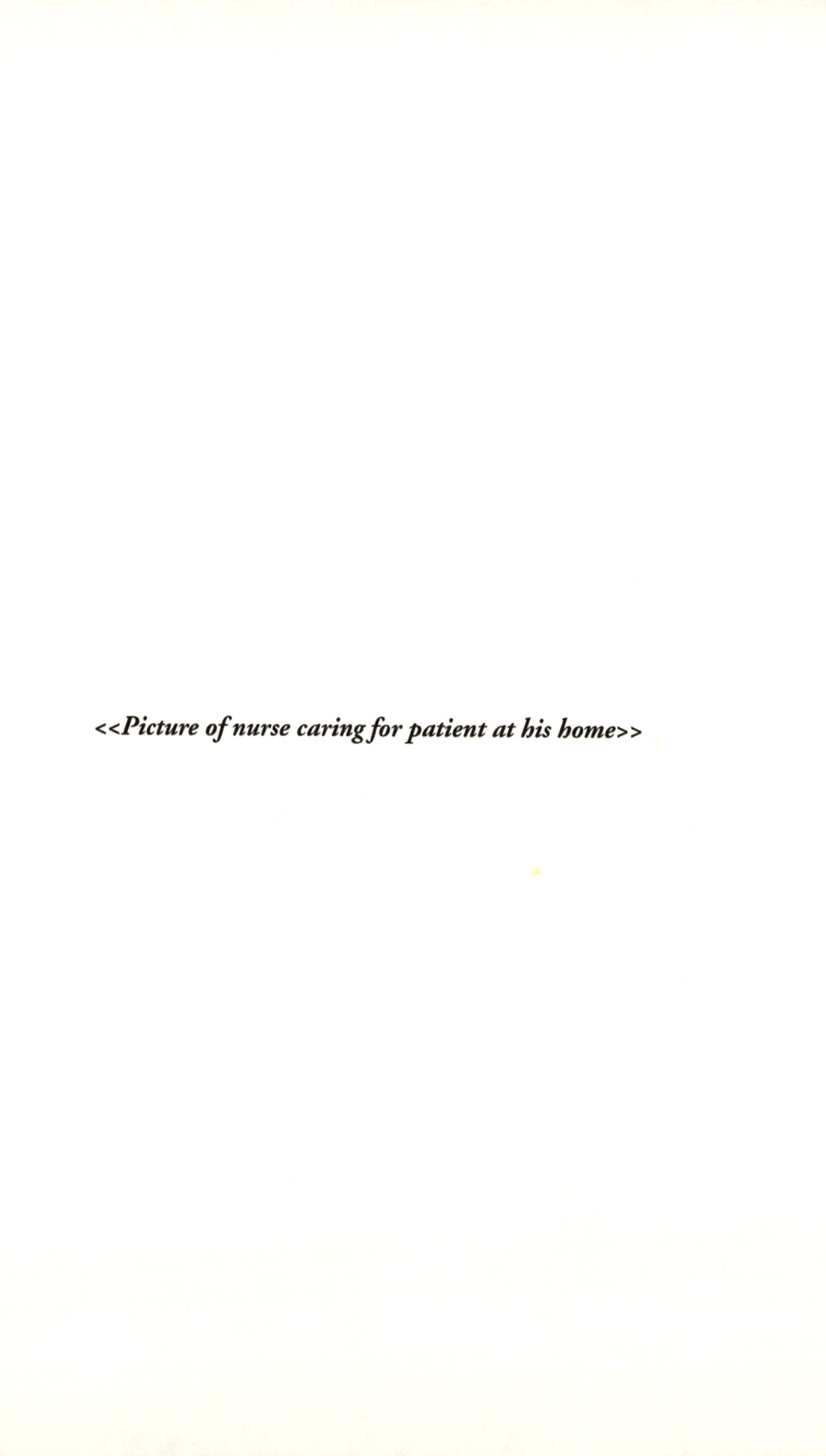

<<Picture of nurse caring for patient at his home>>

EXPERIENCED COMMUNITY NURSING FIRSTHAND

Carmen Alicea, RN, MSN, WCC

Why Nursing?

HAVING THE QUALITY of a giving person, being empathetic, and having the will and power to assist others are some of my reasons for becoming a nurse, working in a hospital and experiencing patients' unfortunate experiences with those nurses, doctors, and facility staff who proudly and without shame express their uncompassionate, unempathetic service.

My Inspiration

I was inspired to share my vast, unique experiences in home care. One would have to walk in my shoes to understand the intangible experience of nursing in the community. Only community nurses can empathize with and understand my experiences. It is a whole world with its unique culture where many lives are touched by a home visit. The various conditions, surroundings, and environments one could not even fathom. Clients in the community need extraordinary care.

Community nursing places nurses in a needed position. Many are unaware or just don't realize the invaluable experience in caring for a client/patient in the community. This book recognizes and reflects the nursing services provided in the home setting.

Nursing has been defined and described in various ways by many different leaders and nursing theorists. Opportunities to care for patients exist in all settings, including the community patient's home. Community nursing will be defined by my firsthand experience in home care—applying nursing practice in the comfort of a patient's environment, setting, surroundings, and a patient's concept of home.

Applying the nursing process in the comfort of a patient's home is a nurse's way of survival within the realm of applying the nursing process in the community setting.

From the inception of becoming a nurse, the nursing process has been assessment, nursing diagnosis, planning, implementation, and evaluation with expectations of a positive outcome.

In the following pages, you will read about the basic process in the nursing profession being applied in the community, the experiences of a home-care nurse's encounters, and how, in the midst of it all, nurses survive the positive with the negative encounters. The amount of time spent in traffic, looking for an address, then looking for a parking space and a patient's home is an experience by itself.

A community nurse plans for each visit as one becomes familiar with each client. The plan does not always take place as planned. Home visits may become habitual; however, it is never a routine. Home-care nurses must be prepared to adjust to any given situation in the community. Home-care nurses become experts in developing individualized relationships, creating the environment of trust, respect, and professional integrity.

Home-visiting nurses have to be creative to save patients' lives, including their own, to apply the nursing process, and to apply holistic nursing in all types of environments. From upscale-living patients who have adequate family support to patients residing below poverty level. Home-care nurses service the middle class with housekeepers to patients with no support system who reside in deplorable conditions—infested with roaches/rats, abuse, and drugs/alcoholism.

The health-care delivery system in the home is diverse and unique. One of the beauties of home care is the multiple cultural backgrounds and its challenges. A visiting home-care nurse has to be culture and gender sensitive. I learned quickly how to adjust to the diverse customs and cultural values and enjoyed the opportunity.

My purpose is to share my experiences in the health-care delivery system in the community. The short stories illustrate actual facts and events. The book talks about the process in providing nursing at the client's home and providing excellent practice.

In the home-care setting, nurses encounter factors beyond the client's physical condition. For example, the environment of care, relationships, spiritual needs, and support systems are crucial to the achievement of positive outcomes. This is especially true when abuse of a client is suspected. When you suspect abuse, you must incorporate the client, family, and caregiver into your total assessment and care plan. When providing home care, one has to use all senses and be an astute listener. Pay careful attention to the client as a whole, his physical appearance, his behavior, his responses, and his body language. Compare the patient's family/caregiver's responses to the patient's responses. Many clients protect the abuser for fear of being left alone or of increased abuse.

In providing home-care nursing service, the nurse has to address all individuals involved, especially the caregiver. If abuse is suspected, it opens up a Pandora's box and creates a high volume of paperwork for the nurse reporting the suspected abuse. It has to be addressed in an interdisciplinary team meeting, which consists of individuals from various disciplines: a social worker, a psychologist, a physical therapist, nurses, managers, and a chaplain. It becomes a cumbersome process. However, for the client's safety, it has to take place.

The nurse as an educator has to educate the patient (if the patient's mental status permits) and the caregiver about many different topics (e.g., nutrition, medication, proper transferring, exercise, hand washing, hygiene, normal limits and out-of-range blood pressure and glucose values, and so on).

The home-visiting nurse's experiences are invaluable experiences in the community. A requirement to being a home-visiting nurse is to place one's health and life on the line, yet the sacrifices go unnoticed.

*   *   *

The names used in this book are fictitious to protect the privacy of the clients. However, the facts are actual events.

Admission Assessment

The admission assessment has to be done by a registered nurse. The nurse has to prepare the client and significant other—be it a family member, friend, or caregiver—for the lengthy process.

The admission assessment consists of a packet with multiple forms to be completed. The admission packet consists of the nursing assessment, which has many, many questions, including the Braden scale, a psychosocial form, a depression tool, the Barthel tool, the Zarit tool, and an environmental form. Part of the admission is a full physical assessment. Many of the questions are personal and insensitive.

I always start by introducing myself, explaining the purpose of my visit, and making the client and significant other aware of the lengthy admission process. Depending on various factors, I may have to divide the admission process into two to three home visits before I can complete the entire admission. At times, the clients become so frustrated with the admission process that they decline service and ask the nurse to leave. It may be in a respectable manner, or it may be simply by attempting to push, yell, or scream curses at the nurse in order to get the nurse out of the home.

Once a patient is admitted into the nursing home-care program, a licensed practical nurse can proceed to follow the case with quarterly registered nurse supervision. Visiting nurses collaborate with the patient's primary care provider, social worker, and other required disciplines to provide a complete health-care delivery system to the client in the comfort of the client's home.

CASE A

THE FIRST CASE I was assigned to was for medication management. Mr. A lived in the Bronx, in a fourth-floor walk-up. I was equipped with my clinical bag and the patient's information: address, list of patient's medication, past medical history. I had already checked the patient's chart and had a vivid picture of Mr. A. The clinical bag contained a stethoscope, thermometer, alcohol swabs, hand sanitizer, soap, pens, pencils, plastic bag, isolation clothing, gloves, scissors, syringes, specimen tube, tourniquet, and educational material on diabetes (DM), hypertension (HTN), infection control, safety, fall, emergency hazards, and heat wave information. The bag also contained a sharps container, glucometer, glucometer supplies, flashlight, gauze, normal saline, tape, and measuring guides. The supplies in the clinical bag are a requirement from the Joint Commission. Whether we need the supplies for the visit or not, the clinical bag has to be supplied according to Joint Commission standards.

Mr. A was an eighty-seven-year-old Hispanic man with HTN, DM, lumbago, and vertigo. He lived alone in a one-bedroom apartment, well furnished, with adequate lighting. When I introduced myself, the patient greeted me with a hug and a kiss on the cheek before I could extend my hand for a handshake. I felt the need to shake his hand, but he looked at me as if something was wrong. I introduced myself and explained the purpose of my visit. Mr. A asked me to follow him to the kitchen and to sit down.

The moment Mr. A opened the door, I started my assessment (the nursing process) by taking note of his clothing and any possible body odor; he had none. Mr. A was very clean. On the way to the kitchen, I continued to assess my surroundings. I noted an altar with lit candles. *He lights candles every evening for his deceased wife.* I noted many throw rugs, a smoke alarm, two televisions, and many radios. I also noted how neat Mr. A maintained his apartment. There were many family pictures and pictures of Jesus Christ. Mr. A enjoyed music and conversation about Puerto Rico and his experiences in the military service (army). I asked if I could wash my hands in the bathroom—of course, part of the plan was to assess the bathroom. Yes, I noted grab bars, a shower chair, and two throw rugs on the floor.

I rejoined Mr. A in the kitchen, showed him my identification, and explained again the purpose of my visit. I told Mr. A that I had to check his medications and his vital signs and skin and ask a few questions. Of course, a few questions consist of the admission assessment, psychosocial form, Zarit tool, geriatric depression tool, Barthel tool, mini-mental tool, and so on. Mr. A said, "My child, ask me anything you like because I think I know those medications more than my own doctor. The first thing I do in the morning is shower, eat a piece of toast, and take my medication with tea." I asked Mr. A who prepares his dinner. Mr. A said, "Listen, child. I cook for myself. I was a chef in the army. I don't need anyone here. I cook, clean, iron, wash my clothes, and go food shopping. All I need is someone to come and sit with me for a few hours to talk about anything and watch the time go by."

I checked his vital signs, which were within normal limits at the time. His blood pressure read 110/64. I asked Mr. A if he knew his baseline. Mr. A stated it was usually the same or lower.

I provided Mr. A with a list of his medications and reviewed the list with him. He was quite informed of all his medications. I informed/reminded him to call 911 in the event of an emergency. I informed Mr. A about infection control and hand washing, as well as the safety hazards in his apartment; for example, the candles could cause a fire and the throw rugs could cause him to fall. I suggested meals-on-wheels to prevent any accidents in the kitchen, such as a fire or the possibility of him getting burned.

I provided two medication pillboxes and prefilled them following the medication list. As I was filling the medication pillboxes, Mr. A asked me what part of Puerto Rico I was from and talked to me in Spanish. He began talking to me about his hometown in Puerto Rico and when and how he first came to live in New York City. He talked about his wife and how he cared for her until she passed on. In fact, Mr. A lights up the candles daily to give light to his wife in her journey of destiny.

I sat and listened, understanding that he was lonely and needed an ear—anyone's ear. He just needed the presence of another human being. I then asked him to sign the consent form indicating that I visited him. Mr. A stated, "You are going already. I haven't finished telling you about my hometown in Puerto Rico." I told Mr. A that next time he could tell me a little more about himself. He then responded, "Well, if you have to go, then go." I explained that I had other visits and promised to stay an extra ten to fifteen minutes on the next visit. I then reminded him about the candles/rugs/infection control and to dial 911 in the event of an emergency. I provided Mr. A with my business card. Mr. A hugged me and kissed my cheek. I allowed it because I understood his culture and was able to sense that he meant no harm. It was part of his culture to greet a female in such a way to express acceptance of the visit.

I was able to apply the first nursing process assessment. I assessed his home, the safety issues at his home, his appearance, the way he ambulated, and his loneliness and need for companionship. Mr. A was mentally sharp. At the age of eighty-seven, he did a lot for himself and was quite independent. From assessing the altar, I knew he was a religious man, believing in the Catholic faith.

This visit went smooth. I cleaned my hands as soon as I got into the car with 70 percent alcohol hand sanitizer.

I then returned to my place of employment to document the visit in a timely manner. On my way to the office, I was thinking about Mr. A. I felt sorry for him. I felt uncomfortable leaving him without finishing his story, but I knew he would always have a story to tell just to keep me there. To have that human touch, the human companion for just a short time.

I started to think about my elderly mother, who resides alone. I called her and talked to her for fifteen minutes. That evening, I called her again. My mother thought something was wrong. I had to explain to her my visit with Mr. A and how I felt and that I hoped she would always call when she felt lonely or in need of talking. My mother sent me her blessing and asked me to pray for the elderly who do not have any family. I then called my mother every day to ask her questions about Puerto Rico and her experience growing up in Puerto Rico. I was searching for information to be able to understand and communicate with Mr. A.

This visit with Mr. A was my initial visit out of many encounters.

*   *   *

CASE B

MY NEXT VISIT was on a Saturday. The visit was for wound-care management. The client was a female veteran known as Mrs. B. She was eighty-four years old, totally dependent, and lived in a fifth-floor walk-up in Harlem. One had to climb four steps to enter the building, but there were two steps missing, and each step was high. The music was loud, and there were many Afro-American men drinking and talking at high volume. The building did not have any lights. One of the men offered to help me with my bag. I felt apprehensive but had no choice but to take the chance. Another man held out his hand to help me up the steps. I must admit that I was concerned but walked through my fear.

I was able to walk up to the fifth floor. There were no lights in the hallway on my way up. I thanked God for the light that came in through the hallway windows. I knocked on the door. A young Afro-American lady answered the door; before I identified myself, the young lady opened the door wide and motioned me to come in. She identified herself as the home health aide (HHA). It was a long corridor before the living room where Mrs. B was sitting. I had to pass a room on the left. I noted garbage on the floor, holes on the walls, and saw something jump. I honestly thought it was a cat, and I said, "Oh, Mrs. B has a cat." The HHA looked with her eyes wide open and said it was a rat. I loudly responded, "What?" The HHA looked at me and said, "A rat." I continued to walk past a bathroom. The bathroom seemed clean with no shower curtains, no towel, no soap, no safety gadgets (e.g., grab bars, shower chair, or long handheld shower head)—only a roll of bathroom tissue. The next room was the kitchen with an old kitchen sink. There were many dirty dishes. I noted a clean plate, a cup, and a spoon set aside. (The clean utensils were the ones the HHA used for Mrs. B.) There was garbage all over the place, roaches, dirty walls, and newspapers on the window in place of a shade or curtains. The lighting was not bright.

I walked into the living room where Mrs. B was sitting watching television. The television had a hanger in place of an antenna. The picture was not clear, and the volume stopped at one medium level. There was also another room with no bedroom doors but with a mattress on the floor and someone sleeping on it. The person sleeping was a male. An Afro-American male.

I looked at Mrs. B, introduced myself, and explained the purpose of my visit. I asked how she was feeling. Mrs. B responded, "Okay. Watching a little bit of television." I asked who was sleeping on the mattress. Mrs. B stated, "I don't know, but it could be one of my neighbors who come and stay with me to make sure I am okay." At that moment, the person jumped up and walked away. He was barefooted and had a stench on him. A few minutes later, he walked back into the living room, changed the channel, and sat next to Mrs. B with a plate of unidentifiable food. He sat quietly and ate. I introduced myself to him, but he would not respond. Mrs. B stated, "Don't mind him. He gets like that sometimes." The person stated, "Do your job and I will do my business." I asked Mrs. B if it was okay that I interview her in the presence of this person. Mrs. B nodded her head in agreement that the person could stay. So I started asking questions. It was difficult for me to concentrate because of the male who sat next to Mrs. B. I looked at the HHA and asked if she was okay. She just nodded in a yes gesture but gave the impression of being afraid.

I checked Mrs. B's vital signs and addressed the pressure ulcer she had on her heels. Mrs. B said it was improving. I noted her bilateral lower extremities were grossly edematous and advised her to elevate her legs as much as possible. I suggested to the HHA to cook with no or low sodium. The HHA nodded in agreement. Mrs. B said, "I never put salt on my food." The unidentified person immediately said, "Stop lying. You know you do. What do you think all that fast food has?" I looked at the HHA and asked if she cooked for Mrs. B. She responded, "I can only warm up and serve what she has in the refrigerator." I asked her about the list of her duties. She provided me a list that indicated that her duties included cleaning, washing clothes for Mrs. B, and running errands. The HHA said, "I am hired to care for Mrs. B, not everyone else. The few dishes you saw clean in the kitchen are the ones I washed. I clean the bathroom, but Mrs. B does not have much. In fact, she has three outfits, and she has all of them on." I asked Mrs. B why she had three outfits on, and she stated, "This way I will not lose them or misplace them." I asked Mrs. B who took care of her finances, to which she responded, "My friends." I asked her how she got to her appointments. Mrs. B responded, "That is why you were sent here, because I cannot walk. But if I have to go anywhere, my friends carry me down the stairs." The unidentified person asked Mrs. B for pain medication. Mrs. B said, "I gave you all I had. I do not have any more." The person grabbed a cloth bag Mrs. B had by her side and looked through the bag for pain medication, threw the bag on Mrs. B's lap, and left the apartment.

I was in no position to say or do anything because it would have made matters worse. After the person left, the HHA said, "Today will be the first and last time I come to work in this place. I am afraid of the rats and the traffic of people coming in and out. In fact, Mrs. B said her friends take her money and buy her fast food, but she never receives any change back, and she is always behind on her bills. According to the last HHA, her lights were turned off, and she has an extension cord outside the window drawing electricity from a streetlamp pole." I informed the home health aide that one of her duties was to report to her supervisor anything out of the norm, including patient abuse. The home health aide stated she was planning on doing so after she leaves Mrs. B's apartment at the end of the work shift.

I addressed Mrs. B and completed the admission assessment. I reviewed her medications and noted there was no oxycodone 10 mg left in the container. Mrs. B was discharged the day before with all her medications, including a supply of ninety tablets of oxycodone 10 mg. I did not bother asking where the rest of the medication (oxycodone 10 mg) was because I assumed her so-called friends took them. I asked her if she was in any pain, and she denied any pain or discomfort. During the entire visit, I did not remove the bag from my shoulders. I explained to Mrs. B about the health and safety hazard in the apartment. I asked if she was interested in a nursing home. She was not a candidate for an assisted living because she was not able to ambulate with the condition of her bilateral extremities. Mrs. B responded, "I am not interested. Thank you. I have my neighbors and friends who look after me. In fact, they will be very upset if I was to leave them."

I informed Mrs. B of her rights as a patient and an elderly person. I had to inform her that I was forced to call Adult Protective Services. Mrs.

B immediately asked me to leave, yelling, "You can call or do whatever you want. I know my rights." I attempted to calm Mrs. B, but it was to no avail. I was not sure if Mrs. B was acting out to protect those she called her friends or for fear of being admitted in a nursing home. I was also aware of the fact that no one likes to leave their home. Mrs. B was used to the environment and felt safe with her friends because they ran her errands to the fast-food places. Mrs. B seemed content with the situation she found herself in. In retrospect, the television and unkempt furniture belonged to her. She did not want to lose her possessions. I informed Mrs. B that she had options to live in better conditions with services. Mrs. B lowered her tone and asked me to leave her home. I left the dilapidated apartment Mrs. B called home.

I made it down the stairs and out the building. I jumped over the missing steps with my clinical bag. One of the fellows standing out there playing the music stated, "She learns fast," referring to me jumping over the missing steps with the clinical bag on my shoulder.

I walked over to an open fire hydrant and washed my hands. I returned to my office and documented. On my way to the office, I prayed for Mrs. B's safety and the safety of all the abused elderly in this world. I wrote an e-mail to the social worker regarding Mrs. B's situation. The social worker addressed the situation by involving Adult Protective Services. Later, I became aware that Mrs. B was assigned a legal guardian who lasted with her a short period due to the deplorable conditions. Mrs. B was then placed in a community nursing home where she passed approximately six months later.

*   *   *

CASE C

I PREPARED TO visit Mr. C at his home in the Bronx, in an area known to be rough—Valentine Avenue and 184th Street. This neighborhood is known to be a busy area with high crime. There always seems to be people sitting in front of the building, loud music, kids running around, teenagers holding on to a chain used as a leash for their dogs, and many loud conversations going on all at the same time. I always dreaded having to come to such an environment. But it is part of the job as a home-care nurse.

I was visiting Mr. C for wound care. Mr. C was a grossly obese patient. Mr. C weighed approximately four hundred pounds. Mr. C remained in bed for most of the time. He rarely left the room except to use the bathroom. A king-size bed and a small dresser with a television on it were the only items that fitted in Mr. C's room. His room was very small. I had to keep my clinical bag on my shoulders at all times. Though it was difficult, I managed to provide wound care—changed the dressing on his left foot. Mr. C was very respectable. I usually found him reading the Bible or watching television.

His wife slept in the living room, which she kept immaculate. She managed everything, from paying the bills to cleaning and cooking. I once saw her serve four pork chops with a mountain of potatoes and collard greens on a huge plate. I asked her if she ate all the food on the plate. Her response was that the plate was for Mr. C. I put on my teaching cap and informed Mrs. C about healthy eating and portions. I went into my clinical bag and handed her pamphlets on the nutritional pyramid. From the look on her face, I knew she was well informed. Mrs. C said, "Listen here. I know about healthy eating, can't you tell? Look at me. But I have to do my wifely duty and serve my husband as he wishes. That is his life. I told him more than a thousand times, but he does not listen. He can't even walk." I asked if Mr. C could cook. Mrs. C's response was, "Picture that." We both shared a smile. I suggested she serve smaller portions and explained the connection between food and one of the patient's diagnoses, diabetes.

Mrs. C removed one of the pork chops and some of the potatoes and asked me to listen. When she walked to Mr. C's room and handed him the plate, he said to her, "You are short one pork chop, and what's up with my potatoes?" Mrs. C said, "Ask the nurse." Mr. C thought I left the apartment and said, "That nurse don't know nothing. She's not the one who's going to stay hungry." To his surprise, I walked into the room and talked to him.

I made several appointments for Mr. C to meet with the dietician, but he never made any of the appointments. Mr. C always had an excuse as to why he could not make the appointments. I suggested exercise. Mrs. C laughed so loud that I joined in her laughter. Then I asked, "What are we laughing about?" Mrs. C said, "Picture that, Mr. C exercising. He can barely walk," and walked out of the room.

I taught Mr. C how to exercise with his arms. Mr. C had an order for daily wound-care dressing. I took this opportunity to exercise with Mr. C using his arms, reaching to the ceiling and down. Mr. C started with three, then progressed to three sets of ten. In a couple of months, Mr. C was walking the hallway outside of his apartment. Mrs. C told me, "You are one special lady. Not even the church pastor could get Mr. C to move a muscle. The only muscle I know Mr. C would constantly work is his jaw muscle." She laughed and went back inside the apartment. Mr. C looked at me and said, "Don't worry, Carmen, we'll show them."

Mr. C walked twice a week, then three times a week. It was not much, but I was proud that I had Mr. C walking and exercising his arms. I used the time we walked to talk to Mr. C. He shared many military stories. Since Mr. C believed in God, I told him that his body was the temple of the Lord and he must not allow the enemy to steer him in the wrong direction. I reminded Mr. C that overeating is gluttony, which is a sin. I dared to say, "Mr. C, you know this. You are a God-fearing man. You know your Bible." At the same time I was talking to Mr. C, I was praying that he did not send me away or become annoyed. Mr. C just listened and nodded his head in agreement.

On one of the visits, Mrs. C said, "Carmen, you better check his temperature. He [referring to Mr. C] asked me to buy orange juice instead of soda and asked for not one but two less pork chops." I felt victorious and smiled. Of course, I had to thank the Lord. I congratulated Mr. C, who smiled and started telling a story about his boot camp training days and how thin he was. On the next visit, Mr. C shared photos of himself when he was in the military.

I became close to Mr. C and Mrs. C. At times, I would bring him bananas or an apple or two. I continued to visit Mr. C until one day I decided to visit extra early to have time for additional visits added to my schedule. There was no music, no crowd in the front of the building, no kids running or playing, no multiple conversations at the same time, and no dogs to fear. I opened the elevator door and was confronted by a black male who was squatting moving his bowels. I was shocked at what I saw. For a moment, I was paralyzed. We both looked at each other, and the man said "excuse me" in a sarcastic manner, letting me know that I was invading his privacy. I then let go of the elevator door and said, "Oh s—t." I walked up the stairs to Mr. C's apartment. While walking up the stairs, I thought, *The nerve of that person. But true, I invaded his privacy.* I did not see any need to share with Mr. C what had occurred, so I went on with my visit as usual.

On another visit to Mr. C, I encountered a loose dog—a pit bull. I ran so fast and climbed on top of a car. I was shaking and peed my pants. Thank God for panty liners. The owner of the dog came after the dog, laughing, and said, "You should not have run, he does not bite." I was speechless. I did not make it to Mr. C's apartment. I walked to the government's vehicle I was assigned and sat for a few minutes. I started to cry, prayed, got myself together, and proceeded to my next visit. I then called Mrs. C and asked if she could change Mr. C's dressing. Mrs. C said, "If he wasn't so big, he could change his own dressing. I'll do it, Carmen. I will not do it like you, but I'll do the best I can."

I e-mailed the doctor and had the order changed to visit Mr. C three times a week. It was difficult, but I did manage to go back. I became used to the stairs and refused to take the elevator. I looked at the positive side; it was an exercise for myself. The wound healed, and the time came to discharge Mr. C. Mr. C had also lost a significant amount of weight. Mr.

C lost forty-five pounds, which made a difference in his breathing and getting around. Mr. C started visiting his neighbors and made some of his appointments. It was difficult to discharge Mr. C because I became fond of Mr. and Mrs. C. I called and sent them Christmas cards until one day I saw Mr. C in the hospital with a diagnosis of congestive heart failure (CHF). Mr. C never made it out the hospital. I contemplated on many occasions to call/visit Mrs. C but never got around to it. I pray the Lord comforts her pain.

*   *   *

CASE D

M R. D WAS an eighty-four-year-old male who resided with his wife in the Bronx. Mrs. D always answered the door. The apartment was always clean and organized. I had to visit Mr. D every two weeks for medication management and to fill two pillboxes. They were pleasant and never had any questions, so I volunteered information and asked many questions.

On one of the visits, Mr. D answered the door. I asked where Mrs. D was. Mr. D pointed to the sofa in the living room and said, "She [referring to his wife] is sleeping. I guess she is tired. She was fixing lunch, then she just laid down to rest." I looked at Mrs. D and asked Mr. D if she had not been well. Mr. D responded, "As far as I know, she is okay. She has not complained about anything. In fact, I believe she's healthy because she never complains about being sick." I had a strange feeling. I went to check her pulse, and immediately Mr. D stated, "Let her rest." I proceeded to check her pulse and noted it was faint. I asked if she had any medical condition— diabetes, hypertension, anything. Mr. D shrugged his shoulders and stated that he did not know.

I noted on the refrigerator door a schedule to take insulin. Mr. D was not on insulin. I pulled out my glucometer and checked Mrs. D's glucose level. The glucometer read 13 mg/dl. Immediately, I called 911 and Mr. D's daughter. I attempted to wake Mrs. D. Mr. D continued to ask me to let her rest. I asked Mr. D if there was any juice. Again, Mr. D shrugged his shoulder and stated that he didn't know. I took the liberty to check the refrigerator, got a small glass of orange juice, and added enough sugar to make a sugar paste. I propped four pillows under Mrs. D's head, placed a spoonful of sugar in her cheek, and rubbed it. In a matter of minutes, Mrs. D opened her eyes and asked me what I was doing. I explained and then informed her that I had called 911 and her daughter. When 911 arrived, I explained what had occurred. They checked Mrs. D's glucose level, which read 182 mg/dl, and had Mrs. D sign a form refusing to go to the hospital. I then called their daughter to inform her that her mother was okay.

Mrs. D talked to her daughter on the telephone and proceeded as if nothing occurred. She opened the icebox and removed a pack of meat to start getting ready for dinner. Mr. D just sat looking at what was happening, not asking or saying anything. He did not understand what went on. I explained to Mr. and Mrs. D what had happened and reeducated them on diabetes, the signs and symptoms, and all the pros and cons I felt they should know. They nodded in agreement and repeated everything in their own words. However, I was not sure Mr. and Mrs. D understood. I then had to address the reason for my visit—assess Mr. D's medication and prepour two pillboxes. Then I called their daughter and suggested for her to get into the habit of calling her parents daily to remind them about their medications and Mrs. D about her finger stick. On the next visit, I attempted to install the health buddy.

The health buddy is an equipment that is installed in the patient's home to monitor the patient remotely. Installing the equipment and attempting to train Mr. and Mrs. D on how to use it was to no avail as they were not interested and did not use it at all. Again, I called their daughter and suggested she remind her father, Mr. D, about answering the health buddy. That did not work either. I ended up removing the health buddy equipment.

On the next three scheduled visits, no one answered the telephone. In fact, no one answered the telephone at the patient's home or at the daughter's home. I mailed a note requesting the daughter to please call my office. I received no response. One day, I decided to visit, and to my surprise, Mr. D answered the door. I asked where his wife, Mrs. D, was, and he said she died a couple of months ago. I extended my condolence. He seemed numbed. I asked if he wanted to attend bereavement groups. He refused and said he was all right. He said he stayed with his daughters over the weekend and had a home health aide helping him with the cleaning and shopping. He said he also receives meals-on-wheels. I completed my visit and left feeling sad for Mr. D. I wish I could do more. I called his daughter who shared what had happened. She stated that when she called her father (Mr. D) and inquired about Mrs. D, Mr. D would say that she was sleeping. This went on for two days until the daughter recalled what

I had shared with her. She then decided to call 911 and went to visit her parents. Emergency rescuers (911) arrived before the daughter to find Mrs. D dead on her bed. Mr. D went with his daughter, who resided in upstate New York for a few weeks before he insisted on returning to the apartment. Mr. D was diagnosed with mild dementia. It turned out that Mrs. D had cervical cancer and did not share it with anyone so as not to worry her family. Mrs. D was a woman who cared for her family and protected them from any unpleasant situation.

*   *   *

CASE E

AT FIRST, VISITING Mr. E was a challenge. There was always a young man standing in the hallway, facing the entrance. He made it obvious he had a gun in his pants. He would not smile or greet me. The young man thought I was the feds because I drove a government vehicle. I started by saying good morning. At first, I was not recognized as someone he should talk to. I once asked the young man to keep an eye on my car so I do not get a ticket. The young man said, "Ticket? You have undercover plates." I smiled and said, "I wish. I am a nurse." I showed him my identification and asked him to please keep an eye on my car. The young man said okay. After several times of greeting this young man, mentioning the weather, and asking him to mind my vehicle, he finally smiled and responded. Before I knew it, I made friends with some of the teenagers who solicited in the neighborhood. Mr. E told me once that the young man asked how his nurse was doing. From then on, I knew I was safe.

Mr. E was a seventy-seven-year-old Hispanic male who resided on a first-floor dilapidated apartment. He lived alone after his wife passed. He had no children and no living relatives. He had rheumatoid arthritis; his fingers were deformed from the arthritis. This made it difficult for Mr. E to care for himself, so he had a home health aide to clean, wash his clothes, and do the shopping. The home health aide omitted the cleaning aspect, and Mr. E was afraid to say anything for fear of losing the aide and not having anyone to talk to or to wash his clothes weekly. He was afraid of being hurt by his neighbors, drug dealers, and drug users that he would allow the drug users to use his bathroom. His neighbors borrowed monies. Mr. E said they would pay him back, but I found that very doubtful. The landlord continued to say Mr. E owed back rent for when Mr. E was hospitalized. Mr. E paid the landlord in cash. The landlord had no records to indicate Mr. E paid for the back rent. The landlord would then come periodically to collect the amount for the back rent. At first, Mr. E would try to remind the landlord that he paid him in cash and did not get a receipt. The landlord said it was impossible and would threaten to evict him Mr. E.

Mr. E paid for the same rent several times. One day, I visited and witnessed the conversation and made sure Mr. E received a receipt for paying the rent. I taught the home health aide how to purchase a money order, fill it out, and mail it on a monthly basis. I also called the landlord and informed him about the violations in the apartment: holes on the walls, windows broken, roaches, rats, no hot water or heat. Mr. E was so afraid of losing his apartment he continued to say it was okay. During the winter months, Mr. E kept the oven on for heat. On one of the visits, Mr. E was sitting outside with the aide getting some fresh air. When we went inside and he opened the door, a rat jumped from on top of the kitchen table to the floor. I screamed so loud one of the drug pushers ran with a gun in his hand and asked what the matter was. When I mentioned what it was, he and Mr. E laughed. I involved Adult Protective Services and social services. Mr. E was then moved to an assisted-living facility. At first, he was upset and insisted on going back to his apartment. After a few weeks, he adapted to the place and lived there until he passed. In visiting Mr. E, I went through so many unpleasant experiences. To share all the experiences would mean to merely write a book about the experiences in visiting Mr. E.

* * *

CASE F

M R. F WAS an eighty-seven-year-old male who resided with his eighty-three-year-old wife and one of their children in a low-income housing project in the Bronx. To enter the building, one had to punch in an assigned code to the apartment. The entrance system seldom worked. I had to wait outside for someone to come into or out of the building so I could enter. On many occasions, it was raining, cold, snowing, or very hot. The apartment had just the essential, but the apartment was always clean. The elevators rarely worked and were filthy with an old stench of urine and garbage. Taking the stairwell meant to walk up six flights of stairs. The condition in the stairwell was worse than the elevators.

Mr. and Mrs. F had twelve children. Unfortunately, ten children out of the twelve were into using drugs, incarcerated, or mentally ill.

Mr. F's home visits were for medication management and proper use of insulin. I had to prepour two pillboxes every two weeks and prefill insulin syringes. One of their sons lived with them. On every visit, the son would say Mr. F was losing his memory and threw away his glucometer and blood pressure monitor. At first, I had the glucometer and blood pressure monitor replaced twice. I asked the patient's wife about the glucometer and the blood pressure monitor. Mrs. E stated, "You know, my son has his needs and he does not work, so he does what he can. I hide the glucometer because I thought it to be more important than the blood pressure monitor, but my son gets crazy when he does not have any money for his needs, and I gave him the glucometer. If I would've not given him the glucometer, he would get angry."

I asked if her son ever hit her and her husband, took their monies, or verbally abused them. Mrs. F immediately stated, "Oh, no. John is a good son. He takes us grocery shopping at the beginning of the month and helps us keep our apartment clean. He just has his needs, and if he does not take care of his needs, he yells crazy things." I asked her if she was afraid of her son and would she like help in removing her son. Mrs. F raised her voice and said, "No, I need John here. I feel safe with him here. John will not allow my husband to raise his voice at me or to hit me as he used to when we lived in Puerto Rico and my children were small. I need John. He is a good boy. I just pray that he gets better."

I had to document and call Adult Protective Services to make sure Mr. and Mrs. F were safe. I also provided Mrs. F with information that would benefit her son if he would read and heed the information. Unfortunately, John (the son) was arrested for burglary and incarcerated. I was able to set up home health services for Mr. and Mrs. F. Mr. F was against the home health aide services because his belief was that as long as he had a wife, she should be able to care for him and the home. Mr. F did not understand that his wife was elderly, managing osteoarthritis, and barely able to walk from the pain on her left knee. Mr. F was verbally abusive to his wife.

On one of the visits, he pointed at his wife and said, "Look at her, she is no good for nothing. She cannot take care of me after I gave her twelve children, worked like a dog for many years, and provided for my family. My wife is stupid, never worked a day in her life." I interrupted Mr. F and reminded him that we are in a different era. I reminded him of how difficult it is to raise one child—imagine twelve. I reminded him of the housework, the cooking, cleaning, washing, making sure the bills get paid, and attending to him as a difficult husband. Mr. F remained silent for a few minutes, got up from his seat, walked over to his wife, and kissed her forehead and said, "I guess the nurse is right. You deserve a break from nothing."

I asked him if he beat his wife. Mr. F looked at me sternly and said, "I raised her since she was fourteen years old. I had to teach her who is the boss of this family. My children know who is the boss. Now, she turned my sons against me, and they threaten to disown me if I hit her. My wife has become someone I don't know anymore. Now she talks back and raises the large cooking spoon at me and says she will hit me back if I hit her. She says she is not afraid of me anymore. I know it is because of my children."

Mrs. F joined our conversation and said, "I am thankful for the twelve children we have together. Mr. F has always been a good provider, but I will no longer take any abuse. We have been married for many years, and I know only one husband. Mr. F knows one wife and many other women—enough is enough."

Mr. F said, "Okay, I am sorry, I love you, and let's live happy." They hugged and addressed me. I suggested counseling, but they refused. I was able to complete my visit that day.

I had to discharge Mr. F from the home visit program because he sustained a fall, fractured his left hip, and never left the hospital.

*   *   *

CASE G

I WAS SCHEDULE to visit Mr. G in place of his nurse who was out for a few days. Mr. G was schizophrenic. He had status post I&D on his back related to an abscess. He was obese, with a large protruding stomach from overeating. He was indeed out of shape. His services were for daily wound care. Mr. G lived in a studio apartment that was untidy and dirty. I introduced myself, and the patient allowed me in his apartment. I took care of the wound dressing on his mid back. Mr. G signed the visiting page, and I left. The next day, Mr. G opened the door and I noted how he was dressed with very tight short pants, no foot wear or shirt. I greeted him and tried to ignore how he was dressed. I did not mention anything. I proceeded to attend to his wound. Mr. G asked me if I liked music because he played and sang at a restaurant known to the community. I told him that I liked jazz music but did not have time for it. I was trying to do my job and run out. I had to stay a few minutes longer to listen to him regarding his music playing and singing.

The next day, I visited as I had been scheduled to do and noted he had on his bed several condoms and several one-dollar bills spread out on the bed. The lights were dimmed. I entered the apartment and greeted him. That day was the first time he had ever locked all three locks on the door. He had a strange smile on his face. I asked him why he locked the door, and he replied that he did not want us to get interrupted. I told him I would feel better if the door was unlocked so I could finish up and move on to my next patient because I had a heavy schedule. Mr. G responded, "We will be done in not time." I was nervous, but tried not to show my emotions. I asked him how he was doing, and he replied, "Feeling better than ever and ready." I asked, "Ready for what?" He looked toward the bed, where he had the condoms and the one-dollar bills. I redirected the conversation and said, "Let's take care of the wound because it is healing nicely." He smiled.

I asked him to go wash his hand in the bathroom and to bring tissue. I was trying to give him things to do so I could open the door and run. He went to wash his hands, which only gave me time to unlock two of the locks on the door. I then reminded him about the tissue. He walked back to the bathroom, stating, "Yes, we will need some tissue to clean up after." I was able to unlock the third lock. I then asked him to let the water from the tub run to get fresh water so I could wash his wound. Mr. G was very cooperative. I was able to run to open the door and ran down the stairs. All I could hear was Mr. G calling my name and asking me to come back. I was so nervous. I sat in the car, said a prayer, and waited until I calmed down.

After returning to the office, I suggested for Mr. G to make an appointment to have his wound evaluated and orders changed to allow the wound to heal without dressing changes. It worked out fine as his wound was healing nicely and did not need any more dressing changes. Mr. G continued to call the office and ask for me. I answered the telephone and informed him that he was fine and would no longer need home-care services. I also informed him that if the doctor felt he needed home-care services, another nurse would visit accompanied by an escort as the policy had been changed. This was not true, but it was the only way I was able to keep Mr. G from calling.

CARMEN ALICEA

CASE H

I WAS SCHEDULED to see Mr. H one early morning. I was accompanied by the social worker to address any social issues the patient might have had. Mr. H had multiple diagnoses with a recent amputation and moved about in a wheelchair. He lived alone in a studio apartment. When I knocked, the patient yelled, "The door is open, come in," so we proceeded to enter. I had my clinical bag on my shoulder ready for the bimonthly visit for medication management and refilling of his medication boxes.

The patient was sitting at the edge of the bed. After the greeting and introduction of the social worker, whom he was familiar with, the patient stated that he had something to show me. He held up a plastic bag and stated he saved the bags so he would have proof of his discovery. To our amazement, it was bedbugs in the plastic bag! Looking closely, we observed bedbugs crawling on the patient as well as his furniture.

We ran out of the apartment. We went straight to the building management office to report our findings. We had to wait as the superintendent was not available at the moment. When he finally met us, we were in front of the building, scratching ourselves without realizing the extent of our scratching or the places we were scratching. We scratched from our heads to our crotch areas. We introduced ourselves to the superintendent and informed him that the bedbug problem had to be addressed. We discussed the problem as we scratched uncontrollably. The superintendent asked us what was wrong, and we reiterated the situation. He was amused and laughed at how bothered we were from what we observed as evidenced by our constant scratching. To shorten the story, the superintendent stated he would address the problem. The medication pillboxes had to be prepared at work and sent to the patient's home.

When I arrived at home, I fully undressed at the door to my apartment and left my clothing outside my door in a plastic bag until a family member came home and discarded the clothes. I did not even think about or cared if any of my neighbors saw me in my underwear. I washed my sneakers in hot water after my family member suggested not to discard the sneakers because they were brand-new. In a conversation with the social worker, I learned that she had done the same thing when she arrived at her home. It was a serious matter, yet we both enjoyed a good laugh at how it affected us and our reaction to the situation.

*   *   *

CASE I

IT WAS A Wednesday afternoon. I recall clearly driving back to the office when I received a call from the secretary asking me to visit one more patient because the patient's family called complaining that the patient's wound dressing had not been changed in days. This case was not assigned to me. I was covering for the nurse who had to leave home on an emergency situation. The secretary provided me with the patient's address and a brief summary of the patient's history. The patient resided in a low-income housing project in the South Bronx. I had a hunch to pull over before heading to the patient's home and remove my jewelry and put my pocketbook in the trunk. I followed my hunch.

The neighborhood appeared peaceful. Given the location of the Bronx, I was surprised. I looked at the high tower (housing project) before me; I blessed myself with the sign of the cross and proceeded. I entered the building, which had a strong stench of urine. I pressed the elevator button, and the doors to the elevator opened. I started to enter when I was pushed into the elevator and against the wall. At the moment, I did not know what to think or say. I can remember the foul smell of old sweat. The person's knee was up against my back. The person with the knee on my back had me in a choke position. He asked me where I was going. At first, I was not sure if I should answer or not until he pressed harder on my lower back with his knee. I told him where I was going. He asked what I had in my bag. I was carrying a clinical bag. I told him documents to interview a patient. He asked me who I was going to see and on what floor. He took my clinical bag and threw it to a second person, whom I heard say to the first, "Check her pockets." The male who had me up against the wall placed his hands in my turtleneck and checked for a chain. I remember feeling his rough, cold hands. I felt violated and hopeless at that moment. The male with the knee up against my lower back stated, "She does not have anything. Not even a chain." Before I could blink, I felt the force of him trying to push me closer to the elevator wall, and then I was suddenly released. I slowly turned around, straightened myself, grabbed my bag, and stared at the doors from the elevator as they closed. My legs felt heavy, and I was afraid to make a move. The elevator moved to a floor; I did not notice what floor it stopped on. I was not sure what to do or say. I felt numb. Two young Afro-American ladies entered the elevator. At first, I looked at them and they looked back at me with a blank face. I then said, "I was almost mugged." One of the girls responded, "Either you get mugged or you don't. What you mean 'almost mugged'?" Then they began to laugh and got off the elevator.

I rode the elevator up and down for a few minutes with mixed emotions and thoughts. I then got a hold of myself and proceeded to the patient's apartment. A young Afro-American man opened the door to the apartment wide open. I looked from where I stood and noticed another Afro-American male. The first male asked, "Are you coming in?" I looked at him, said yes, and walked in. I asked him not to close the door. He asked me why. I told him that I felt comfortable if the door was kept open. He looked at me as if I was weird. I did not know what to say or do for a couple of minutes, and the male who opened the door asked, "Can we help you?" I then focused my vision, introduced myself, and wondered if they were the two males in the elevator. I was fighting with my thoughts. Suddenly, I felt a wind of strength and asked to see the patient, who was lying in a hospital bed. The second individual stated, "A doctor came this afternoon and saw my dad [referring to the patient]. The doctor said not to change the dressing until he [the doctor] comes back in two days." I called the office, but the answering machine came on. I asked if one of them could sign an encounter form indicating I visited. The male who opened the door asked me if I was okay because my hands were shaking. I thought I was under control, but I realized I was not. I was hesitant to move. I left the apartment and was not sure how to exit—taking the elevator where I was attacked or the stairwell. I peeked at the stairwell, and the stench of urine made the decision for me to pray and take the elevator. I rode the elevator.

I got into the government's car and called my brother. I told my brother about what had just occurred. My brother asked me where I was. After I told my brother my location, my brother demanded I leave the area immediately. My brother suggested I do not bother calling the cops because I would be just a report, a statistic, and nothing would come out of my report. I obeyed my brother, returned the government's vehicle, and went home. I was in a state of shock. My brother came over to console me. He advised me not to enter housing projects alone ever again. The next day, I went to work, typed up a report of contact describing my ordeal, and handed it in. I was informed later in the year by one of my coworkers that my supervisor did not believe my story.

*   *   *

My colleagues and I would return to the office from a long and interesting day in the community as visiting nurses. We would share our experiences and agreed to using the buddy system for certain visits.

I will refer to my colleagues as Nurse 1, Nurse 2, and so on.

*   *   *

Nurse 1

Nurse 1 visited one of her patients who was on antidepressant and other psychotropic medications. The patient was fifty-six years old, a Vietnam veteran who resided with his wife in a one-bedroom apartment. Nurse 1 visited the patient for medication management. Nurse 1 stated that, as usual, they sat at the living room past the kitchen. They sat, and Nurse 1 was able to check his vital signs and ask a few questions when suddenly the patient got up and walked to the kitchen. Nurse 1 stated that she heard fumbling of utensils, got up, and walked toward the kitchen when she was confronted by the patient with a knife in his hand. She stated that the patient went toward her with the knife. Nurse 1 ran toward the door and was able to get away. She had left one shoe behind and her clinical bag. She had to call the police to retrieve her shoe and clinical bag. Emergency rescuers (911) were called, and the patient was taken to the hospital to be treated. It appeared the patient was not compliant with his medications and had a drawback. This was one of the visits continued with a buddy system.

Nurse 2

Nurse 2 visited a patient in Upper Manhattan. This particular patient was known to all the nurses in the visiting program. He was seventy-six years old and lived in a six-room apartment, which was crowded with all types of things he hoarded. The neighborhood was quiet during the morning hours. The parked cars were BMWs, Mercedes-Benzes, Lexuses, etc., with license plates from out of state. The building was well maintained. It was rarely when the elevator was not working. The patient's apartment was on the second floor.

Nurse 2 visited for medication management and to prefill insulin syringes. Nurse 2 visited this patient in the evening hours. She completed her visit and walked outside the apartment to find herself in the midst of gunshots. Nurse 2 stated that she did not run but dove back into the patient's apartment, locked the door, and ran to the back of the apartment with the patient. Nurse 2 was so nervous she could not think to call the police. The patient told Nurse 2 to calm down and wait. The patient stated, "This is not the first time. Those people fighting outside will not harm me because I have been here for many years and mind my own business." The nurse waited for a long while before the patient told her it was safe to leave. Nurse 2 was jolted. The patient had warned the nurse not to call the police; otherwise, the patient would be in danger. Weeks later, another shoot-out occurred with police involved. This incident made the news.

Nurse 3

Nurse 3 was assigned to a patient who was not able to continue to make his appointments for weekly Epogen injections. Nurse 3 had to service the patient outside the apartment. This patient was a hoarder, and there was no space to walk in the apartment. Nurse 3 stated that all one could see was a trail to a filthy bathroom. The patient was sleeping sitting up in a chair. He received meals-on-wheels. The smell was unbearable. Adult Protective Services was involved, the apartment cleaned, but all to no avail. The apartment was back to its previous deplorable condition in a matter of a month. The patient was provided with the option to maintain the apartment in an approachable living manner or make weekly visits to the hospital for the injections. The patient refused to do both. For the safety of the patient, Nurse 3 had to provide services in the hallway outside the apartment. This went on until the patient became too ill to open the door. The police were called, and the patient was transferred to the hospital, then to a nursing home.

*   *   *

The Forgotten

The caregivers are many times forgotten. Caregivers are the nurse's assistant in the home. The caregivers are the ones who communicate to the nurses; they are the eyes and hands of the nurse. The caregivers are the ones who experience everything the patient experiences. The caregivers are empathizers. They are the wives, common-law wives, girlfriends, sons, daughters, extended family members, and many times, just friends or neighbors. Caregivers either are trained by a nurse to care for a patient or learn on their own how to care for the patient. The caregivers make certain the patient takes his medications. They cook, feed the patient, clean up vomits and feces, change adult diapers, dress the patient, and accompany the patient to follow-up appointments.

As community nurses, we address all in the household, including the caregivers. Community nurses have met caregivers who actually care and have committed their time to caring for the patient. There are occasions when the nurse just sits and listens to the caregiver, sets time aside to teach the caregiver, or refers the caregiver to counseling. But community nurses have also met caregivers who are abusers and who neglect the patient. Caregivers who are in for what they can get, for what is beneficial to them. The community nurse has to address both types of caregivers: the caring and the uncaring. In order for the nurse's profession and clinical skills to be acknowledged by the caregivers, the nurse has to establish respect, trust, and develop a positive rapport. Caregivers are an important component to the community nurse.

A high volume of patients/clients require nursing care in the comfort of a familiar environment—their home setting. Therefore, community nurses continue to be the forerunners in health promotion and disease prevention, as well as providing nursing services in the home setting. In providing nursing care in a home setting, community nurses encounter various experiences that should not go unrecognized but often do.

The positive of home care is that the visiting nurse gets to work autonomously, is able to arrange the work schedule, and is able to see the patient in a different environment—his or her home. Seeing the patient in his or her home is a different perspective, and it becomes a true reality. It is rewarding and a satisfying one-on-one experience. The experiences shared here are only a few in comparison to the multitude of parables visiting nurses experience to be shared that are beyond believable.

The following are some of the forms one has to complete during a home visit: Barthel, Zarit, MMSE, admission form, which consists of several pages, and psychosocial and advance directive forms. This is just to mention a few out of all the paperwork entailed in visiting a patient at his or her home.

*   *   *

FORMS

Barthel

Patient Name: _____ Rater: _____ Date: / /	
Activity	Score
Feeding 0 = unable 5 = needs help cutting, spreading butter, etc., or requires modified diet 10 = independent	0 5 10
Bathing 0 = dependent 5 = independent (or in shower)	0 5
Grooming 0 = needs help with personal care 5 = independent, face/hair/teeth/shaving (implements provided)	0 5
Dressing 0 = dependent 5 = needs help but can do about half unaided 10 = independent (including buttons, zips, laces, etc.)	0 5 10
Bowels 0 = incontinent (or needs to be given enemas) 5 = occasional accident 10 = continent	0 5 10
Bladder 0 = incontinent, or catheterized and unable to manage alone 5 = occasional accident 10 = continent	0 5 10
Toilet Use 0 = dependent 5 = needs some help, but can do something alone 10 = independent (on and off, dressing, wiping)	0 5 10
Transfers (bed to chair and back) 0 = unable, no sitting balance 5 = major help (one or two people, physical), can sit 10 = minor help (verbal or physical) 15 = independent	0 5 10 15
Mobility (on level surfaces) 0 = immobile or < 50 yards 5 = wheelchair independent, including corners, > 50 yards 10 = walks with help of one person (verbal or physical) > 50 yards 15 = independent (but may use any aid; for example, stick) > 50 yards	0 5 10 15
Stairs 0 = unable 5 = needs help (verbal, physical, carrying aid) 10 = independent	0 5 10
TOTAL (0–100)	_____

Zarit Assessment Tool

Caregiver's name: _____ Date: _____

The following questions reflect how people sometimes feel when they are taking care of another person. After each question, circle how often you feel that way: never, rarely, sometimes, frequently, or nearly always. There are no right or wrong answers.

	Never	Rarely	Sometimes	Frequently	Nearly always
1. Do you feel that your relative asks for more help than he or she needs?	0	1	2	3	4
2. Do you feel that because of the time you spend with your relative, you do not have enough time for yourself?	0	1	2	3	4
3. Do you feel stressed between caring for your relative and trying to meet other responsibilities for your family or work?	0	1	2	3	4
4. Do you feel embarrassed over your relative's behavior?	0	1	2	3	4
5. Do you feel angry when you are around your relative?	0	1	2	3	4
6. Do you feel that your relative currently affects your relationship with other family members or friends in a negative way?	0	1	2	3	4
7. Are you afraid about what the future holds for your relative?	0	1	2	3	4
8. Do you feel your relative is dependent on you?	0	1	2	3	4
9. Do you feel strained when you are around your relative?	0	1	2	3	4
10. Do you feel your health has suffered because of your involvement with your relative?	0	1	2	3	4
11. Do you feel that you do not have as much privacy as you would like, because of your relative?	0	1	2	3	4
12. Do you feel that your social life has suffered because you are caring for your relative?	0	1	2	3	4
13. Do you feel uncomfortable about having friends over, because of your relative?	0	1	2	3	4
14. Do you feel that your relative seems to expect you to take care of him or her, as if you were the only one he or she could depend on?	0 0	1 1	2 2	3 3	4 4
15. Do you feel that you do not have enough money to care for your relative, in addition to the rest of your expenses?	0	1	2	3	4
16. Do you feel that you will be unable to take care of your relative much longer?	0	1	2	3	4
17. Do you feel you have lost control of your life since your relative's illness?	0	1	2	3	4
18. Do you wish you could just leave the care of your relative to someone else?	0	1	2	3	4
19. Do you feel uncertain about what to do about your relative?	0	1	2	3	4
20. Do you feel you should be doing more for your relative?	0	1	2	3	4
21. Do you feel you could do a better job in caring for your relative?	0	1	2	3	4
22. Overall, how burdened do you feel in caring for your relative?	0	1	2	3	4

Total score: _____

SCORING KEY:
0 to 20 = little or no burden; 21 to 40 = mild to moderate burden; 41 to 60 = moderate to severe burden; 61 to 88 = severe burden.

Screening Tool: The Mini-Mental State Examination (MMSE)

Patient _____ Examiner _____ Date _____

Maximum	Score	
		Orientation
5		• What is the (year) (season) (date) (day) (month)?
5		• Where are we (state) (country) (town) (hospital) (floor)?
		Registration
3		• Name 3 objects: 1 second to say each. Then ask the patient all 3 after you have said them. Give 1 point for each correct answer. Then repeat until he/she learns all 3. Count trials and record. Trials _____
		Attention and Calculation
5		• Serial 7's. 1 point for each correct answer. Stop after 5 answers. Alternatively spell "world" backward.
		Recall
3		• Ask for the 3 objects repeated above. Give 1 point for each correct answer.
		Language
2		• Name a pencil and watch.
1		• Repeat the following "No ifs, ands or buts."
3		• Follow a 3-stage command: "Take a paper in your hand, fold it in half and put it on the floor."
1		• Read and obey the following CLOSE YOUR EYES.
1		• Write a sentence.
1		• Copy the design shown.

_____ **Total Score**

ASSESS level of consciousness along a continuum _____

Alert Drowsy Stupor Coma

"Mini-Mental State." A Practical Method for Grading the Cognitive State of Patients for the Clinician. *Journal of Psychiatric Research*, 12(3): 189-198, 1975. Used with permission.

more information on reverse ➤

GLOSSARY

Barthel index: Consists of ten items that measure a person's daily functioning, specifically the activities of daily living and mobility. The items include feeding, moving from wheelchair to bed and back, grooming, transferring to and from a toilet, bathing, walking on level surface, going up and down stairs, dressing, continence of bowels and bladder. The assessment can be used to determine a baseline level of functioning and can be used to monitor improvement in activities of daily living over time.

Home Health Aide (HHA): An individual who provides services to the client. Services are not limited to maintaining the client's home, assisting the client with taking meds, monitoring vital signs, etc.

I&D: Incision and drainage.

Mini-Mental State Examination (MMSE): The most commonly used test for complaints of memory problems or when a diagnosis of dementia is being considered and is carried out by a medical professional.

Zarit assessment tool: A twenty-two item questionnaire to measure caregiver's burden. The tool was created by Zarit, Reever, and Bach-Peterson in 1980. Each item on the interview is a statement that the caregiver is asked to endorse using a five-point scale. Response options range from 0 (never) to 4 (nearly always).

REFERENCES

Hérbert, R., G. Bravo, and M. Préville. 2000. "Reliability, Validity, and Reference Values of the Zarit Burden Interview for Assessing Informal Caregivers of Community-Dwelling Older Persons with Dementia." *Canadian Journal on Aging* 19: 494-507.

Lai, D. W. L. 2007. "Validation of the Zarit Burden Interview for Chinese Canadian Caregivers. *Social Work Research* 31: 45-53.

Mahoney, F. I., and D. W. Barthel. 1965. "Functional Evaluation: The Barthel Index." *Maryland State Medical Journal* 14: 2.

van der Putten, J. J. M. F., J. C. Hobart, J. A. Freeman, and A. J. Thompson. 1999. "Measuring the Change in Disability after Inpatient Rehabilitation: Comparison of the Responsiveness of the Barthel Index and Functional Independence Measure." *Journal of Neurology, Neurosurgery, and Psychiatry* 66 (4): 480-484.

Zarit, S. H., K. E. Reever, and J. Back-Peterson. 1980. "Relatives of the Impaired Elderly: Correlates of Feelings of Burden." *The Gerontologist* 20: 649-655.

INDEX

A

abuse, 10-11, 19, 33, 43
admission assessment, 12, 14, 19
admission process, 12
Adult Protective Services (APS), 19-20, 32, 42
Alicea, Carmen, 3-4, 9-10, 12, 14, 16, 18, 20, 22-24, 26, 30, 32, 36, 38, 40, 42

B

Barthel Index, 44-45, 49, 51
blood pressure monitor, 31
Braden scale, 12
Bronx, 13, 21, 25, 31, 39
buddy system, 41

C

caregivers, 11-12, 43, 49, 51
community nurses, 5, 9-10, 43

D

depression, 12
diabetes (DM), 13, 22, 25-26

E

emergency hazards, 13
Epogen, 42
experiences, 7, 9-11, 14, 16, 30, 41, 43-44

G

glucometer, 13, 25, 31

H

home care, 9-11, 44
home health aide (HHA), 17-19, 26, 29-30, 49
home health services, 32
hypertension (HTN), 13, 25

I

infection control, 13-15
insulin, 25, 31

J

Joint Commission, 13

L

lumbago, 13

M

Manhattan, Upper, 42
meals-on-wheels, 26
medication management, 13, 25, 31, 37, 41-42
medications, 11, 14, 19, 26, 41, 43
Mr. A, 13-16, 24, 26, 31-32
Mr. C, 21-24, 26-27
Mr. D, 25-26, 29-30
Mrs. B, 17-20
Mrs. C, 21-24, 26-27

N

911 (emergency services), 14-15, 25, 27
nurse, 8-12, 22, 29, 32, 35-36, 39, 41-44
Nurse I, 41
Nurse II, 42
Nurse III, 42
nursing, 9
nursing assessment, 12
nursing home care program, 12
nursing process, 10, 13, 15
nursing services, 9, 43

O

oxycodone, 19

P

pain medication, 19
patient, 8-13, 19, 26, 35, 37, 39-44
physical assessment, 11-12
police, 41-43
primary care provider, 12
psychosocial form, 12, 14

S

safety gadgets, 17
safety hazards, 14, 19, 45
social services, 30
social worker, 11-12, 20, 37-38

V

vertigo, 13

W

wound care, 21

Z

Zarit tool, 12, 14

www.ingramcontent.com/pod-product-compliance
Lightning Source LLC
Chambersburg PA
CBHW021926170526
45157CB00005B/2199